ORAL MORPHINE
Information for patients, families and friends

Robert G. Twycross
MA, DM, FRCP

Macmillan Clinical Reader in Continuing Care
Nuffield Department of Clinical Medicine
John Radcliffe Hospital, Oxford, England

Honorary Consultant Physician
Sir Michael Sobell House
The Churchill Hospital, Oxford, England

Sylvia A. Lack
MB, BS

Director, Chronic Pain Program and Attending Physician
Gaylord Hospital, Wallingford, Connecticut, USA

Consultant in Hospice Care
St Mary's Hospital, Waterbury, Conn., USA

Attending Physician
World War II Memorial Hospital, Meriden, Conn., USA

BEACONSFIELD PUBLISHERS LTD
Beaconsfield, Bucks, England

First published in Great Britain 1988

This book is copyright under the Berne Convention. All rights are reserved. Apart from any fair dealing for the purpose of private study, research, criticism or review, as permitted under the Copyright Act 1956, no part of this publication may be reproduced, stored in a retrieval system, or transmitted, in any form or by any means, electronic, electrical, chemical, mechanical, optical, photocopying, recording or otherwise, without the prior permission of the copyright owner. Enquiries should be addressed to the Publishers at 20 Chiltern Hills Road, Beaconsfield, Bucks, HP9 1PL, England.

American edition © Robert G. Twycross and Sylvia A. Lack, 1987

British edition © Robert G. Twycross and Sylvia A. Lack, 1988

British Library of Cataloguing in Publication Data
Twycross, Robert G.
 Oral Morphine: information for patients, families and friends
 1. Morphine 2. Oral medication
 I. Title II. Lack, Sylvia A.
 616'.0472 RM666.M8
 ISBN 0-906584-22-1

Phototypeset by Gem Graphics, Trenance, Mawgan Porth, Cornwall in 10½ on 12 point Times.
Printed in Great Britain at the University Press, Oxford.

Preface

In recent years a lot has been written about the use of morphine to treat pain in cancer. In this booklet, we have set out to answer a number of questions that patients and their families often ask about this type of treatment. It is more for dipping into, rather than for reading straight through from beginning to end.

For many people morphine has a reputation as a drug of addiction. But the world of the addict and the world of the cancer patient in pain are poles apart. There is no comparison. Injecting drugs into a vein to achieve a 'high' is quite distinct from the regular use of morphine by mouth to relieve pain. Accordingly, we hope that the information given here will set minds at rest, and help to allow the better use of one of the more important cancer pain relief drugs.

The same range of issues are discussed in *Oral Morphine in Advanced Cancer* (Beaconsfield 1984). The warm reception given to this earlier publication for doctors and nurses encouraged us to proceed to present one for patients and families. A question-and-answer approach is used in both. We are most grateful to Mrs Alison Charles-Edwards, SRN, HV, for preparing the initial list of questions for this one, and to several colleagues who gave helpful advice.

We would like to acknowledge with thanks our indebtedness to the Lisa Sainsbury Foundation for financial support towards the publication of this British edition.

Robert G. Twycross
Sylvia A. Lack

Contents

	page
PREFACE	iii
SETTING THE RECORD STRAIGHT ABOUT PAIN IN CANCER	1
COMMON QUESTIONS ABOUT MORPHINE	2
• What is morphine and how does it work?	2
• Morphine? Does that mean I am at the end of the road?	2
• Doesn't morphine speed things up – make you die sooner?	2
• Will morphine take the pain away completely?	2
• If I take morphine now, will there be anything stronger for me when the pain gets worse?	3
• Wouldn't it be better to keep off morphine until things become really unbearable?	3
• Will I need bigger and bigger doses to control the pain?	4
• How long can I go on taking morphine? Does the effect wear off eventually?	4
• Will I become addicted?	4
• Why is morphine given in solution? What about morphine tablets?	5
STARTING TREATMENT WITH MORPHINE	5
• Now that I am starting morphine, what are the important things I need to know about it?	5
• How do you decide how much morphine I need?	6
• What if the starting dose does not completely relieve my pain?	6
• Why every four hours? Wouldn't it make more sense if I just take the morphine when the pain begins to come back?	6
• What should I do if I get behind with my medication?	7
• How soon will I become pain-free?	8
• What about the nights? Do I need to set my alarm clock for 2 a.m.?	8
• A double dose at bedtime? Isn't that a bit dangerous?	8

- Why do I have to take it so often? Couldn't I have a stronger mixture and take it less often? ... 9
- Will I need to use other pain relief drugs with morphine? ... 9
- What will happen to me if morphine does not relieve my pain? ... 10
- Does it matter when I take the morphine in relation to my meals? ... 10
- Is there anything I can add to make the morphine solution taste better? ... 10
- Will I be able to drive the car if I am taking morphine? ... 11

WORKING THROUGH ANY UNWANTED SIDE EFFECTS ... 12

- Doesn't morphine have a lot of side effects? ... 12
- Will I need medication to counteract nausea and vomiting? ... 12
- Will I have to go on taking the anti-vomiting drugs? ... 13
- Will I get drowsy on morphine? ... 13
- Will I go on feeling drowsy or drugged? ... 13
- Will I get confused? ... 14
- Will I get dizzy? ... 14
- What about constipation? ... 14
- I find I've been sweating a lot since I started the morphine. Is this connected? ... 15
- What happens if I am allergic to morphine? ... 15

STILL MORE QUESTIONS ABOUT MORPHINE ... 16

- Why morphine? I thought that was for pain, but my problem is shortness of breath. ... 16
- Is oral morphine really effective? ... 16
- Is it necessary to give more morphine by mouth than by injection? ... 16
- Wouldn't injections be better? ... 16
- Are injections ever needed? ... 17
- Once on injections, is it possible to change successfully to the oral route? ... 17
- Can morphine be given by suppository? ... 17
- Why do some people need more morphine than others? ... 17
- What about the Brompton cocktail? ... 18
- Is diamorphine better than morphine? ... 18
- Why do they create such a fuss about giving morphine in hospital? If there is only one registered nurse on duty, I often have to wait ages until another one comes from the next ward. ... 18

QUESTIONS FROM A RELATIVE OR CLOSE FRIEND   19

- Will it say on the bottle that it's morphine?   19
- Is it necessary to keep the morphine locked up?   19
- Is it all right to keep the bottle of morphine with the other medicines?   19
- Will the morphine mix all right with his other medicines?   20
- Since he has had the pain his appetite has gone completely. Will the morphine help him to eat better?   20
- Will she be safe looking after the baby if she is taking morphine?   20
- What about signing legal documents while taking morphine?   21
- What should I do if he insists on having more than he has been prescribed? Could it kill him?   21
- Is there a danger that she will use the morphine to commit suicide?   22
- If he has no pain and refuses to take the next dose, do I insist on him taking it?   22
- If she becomes unconscious, should the morphine be discontinued?   22

A BROADER VIEW   23

USEFUL ADDRESSES   24

SETTING THE RECORD STRAIGHT ABOUT PAIN IN CANCER

Cancer is relatively common. Possibly one in four of us will develop a cancer at some stage in our lives. Of those who do, only one in four will be completely cured. The rest have to go on living with their cancer until one day it beats them – or they die of something else.

Many patients with cancer develop pain in one or more parts of their bodies, *but not all*. In fact, only two-thirds of patients with widespread cancer have pain. In some it is relieved by anti-cancer treatment and never recurs. In others it persists. You do not, however, have to suffer continuous unrelieved severe pain. And for those who are dying, *a pain-free death is a realistic goal*.

The World Health Organization has recently published a small book entitled *Cancer Pain Relief*. Among the views expressed are the following:
- Cancer pain can and must be treated.
- Drugs usually give good relief, provided the right drug is taken in the right dose at the right time intervals.
- For persistent pain, the drugs should be taken regularly 'by the clock' and not 'as required'.
- The key pain relief drugs are aspirin, codeine and morphine.
- Morphine and morphine-like drugs are the mainstay of therapy for severe cancer pain. Morphine is simple to administer, is widely available and, when properly used, provides good pain relief in most patients.

The World Health Organization document also stresses that it may be necessary to use a second drug with morphine to achieve adequate pain relief. This emphasizes that, although morphine is the mainstay of treatment, it is not the whole answer. Other symptoms may also need to be treated. In addition, most patients and families need the active support of a doctor and a nurse to achieve the best long-term results.

COMMON QUESTIONS ABOUT MORPHINE

1. **What is morphine and how does it work?**

   Morphine is a naturally-occurring substance obtained from the juice of the opium poppy. Codeine comes from the same source. Both substances are effective in relieving pain, cough and diarrhoea. Morphine is a stronger pain-killer and tends to be reserved for when codeine (or a similar drug) fails to relieve pain. Morphine and codeine ease pain by acting on pain centres in the brain and spinal cord.

2. **Morphine? Does that mean I am at the end of the road?**

   Many patients need morphine before and after a major operation, in childbirth, or after a heart attack. In these circumstances, the use of morphine clearly does *not* mean that the person is about to die. It is important that the reason for the use of morphine in cancer is fully understood. Morphine is used to control pain which no longer responds to codeine or a similar drug. It is used at many different stages of the illness, and not just at the end of the road.

   Some cancer patients never need morphine. Many need it for weeks, months or years because of continuing pain. Others need it for just a few days or weeks – perhaps when very ill and close to death.

3. **Doesn't morphine speed things up – make you die sooner?**

   There is no evidence that this is so. Over the years, we have seen many patients take on a new lease of life when free of pain and able to sleep comfortably through the night. Freed from the nightmare of never-ending pain, a patient can take a renewed interest in food, and in life more generally.

4. **Will morphine take the pain away completely?**

   In many cases yes. Relief, however, may well be incomplete with:
   - Bone pain.
   - Neuralgia (nerve pain).
   - Bedsore pain.

Common Questions About Morphine

Though even with these, many patients have excellent results with morphine.

Certain pains should not be treated with morphine at all. For example:
- Burning and stabbing pain caused by nerve damage.
- Muscle spasm pain.
- Tendonitis and arthritis.
- Tension headache and migraine.

Other remedies exist and will, we hope, be recommended by your doctor.

5. If I take morphine now, will there be anything stronger for me when the pain gets worse?

The first thing to get straight is that the pain may never get worse. If it does, an increase in the dose of morphine will control the pain again. This may be a permanent increase, but many patients find they can reduce the dose again later. This frequently happens, for example, after a course of radiation therapy to a painful bone.

Second, there is no need for anything stronger because there is no upper limit to the dose of morphine you can take. In fact, few patients ever need more than 200mg by mouth every 4 hours, and most are well controlled on much lower doses (60mg or less).

If a new pain develops that does not respond to morphine, other treatments can be tried.

6. Wouldn't it be better to keep off morphine until things become really unbearable?

It sounds as if you are worried that your body will 'get used' to morphine and then there will be nothing left to relieve the pain. This does not happen. If a pain returns while you are taking morphine, control will be regained by increasing the dose.

Oral Morphine

7. **Will I need bigger and bigger doses to control the pain?**

   Studies have shown that the dose of morphine usually increases over a period of time. However, these same studies show that the longer someone is on morphine therapy:
   - The rate at which the dose rises is slower.
   - The intervals between dose increases are longer.
   - The chance that the dose will be reduced is greater.
   - The chance of stopping morphine altogether is greater.

8. **How long can I go on taking morphine? Does the effect wear off eventually?**

   If you need morphine you will be able to go on taking it with good effect for the rest of your life, whether this is months or years.

   Normally, the effect does not wear off. The most common reason for an increase in dose is not so much that the morphine effect is wearing off, but that the cancer is causing more pain.

9. **Will I become addicted?**

   What most people mean by this is, 'Will I become hooked and unable to stop the morphine, even if I no longer need it for pain control?' The answer is a simple but definite 'No!' Over the years, we have treated several thousand cancer patients with morphine. We have never had trouble stopping treatment because of 'addiction'. However, you should not stop taking morphine suddenly and completely. If you no longer need morphine for pain control, the dose can be reduced step by step under your doctor's supervision.

   The reason for a gradual reduction in dose is because people who have taken morphine regularly for several weeks usually develop 'physical dependence'. This is not the same as addiction but it does mean that, if morphine is stopped suddenly and completely, withdrawal symptoms would develop.

   There is, however, no medical reason for stopping morphine therapy suddenly and completely. If your pain lessens because of radiation therapy, the morphine will be reduced over several weeks. Moreover,

Starting Treatment With Morphine

the amount needed to prevent withdrawal symptoms is only about one-quarter of the previously used pain-relieving dose of morphine. This means, for example, after a successful injection to deaden a painful nerve, it is possible to reduce the dose of morphine considerably and immediately – and to continue reducing the dose more slowly after that – *without any upset at all.*

10. **Why is morphine given in solution? What about morphine tablets?**

    Morphine is often given in solution because it is easy to swallow and the dose can easily be adjusted. Solutions are readily prepared in different concentrations. If unflavoured, you can add your choice of fruit juice or other liquid to mask the bitter taste of the morphine.

    Morphine tablets are available. If you are still at work you may find tablets more convenient than a bottle of medicine. Long-acting tablets (MST-Continus) usually need to be taken only twice a day.

STARTING TREATMENT WITH MORPHINE

11. **Now that I am starting morphine, what are the important things I need to know about it?**
    - Morphine by mouth (as a solution or tablet) is usually the best way to take it.
    - Solutions should be taken regularly every four hours.
    - Long-acting tablets are usually taken every 12 hours.
    - The dose will be adjusted to meet your individual need.
    - The main side effects are constipation and vomiting; these can be treated effectively.
    - You may need other drugs and treatments as well as morphine.
    - Your response to morphine must be carefully monitored, particularly during the first few weeks.

Oral Morphine

12. How do you decide how much morphine I need?

Most patients starting morphine regularly by mouth have previously been taking codeine (or a similar drug). In most instances, a patient will be changed to 10mg of morphine sulphate solution every four hours.

Occasionally a smaller 'test' dose is recommended in the very elderly or very frail. Sometimes, you will be advised to take an extra 10mg after two hours if the first dose fails to give adequate pain relief, and then to continue on, say, a 15mg dose until reviewed the next day.

On the other hand, if you have been on an alternative to morphine, the starting dose will be higher, possibly 30mg or even 60–100mg.

13. What if the starting dose does not completely relieve my pain?

Don't worry. If you obtain some relief with the starting dose your doctor knows your pain is responsive to morphine. The aim is to increase the dose step by step until your pain is fully relieved. You should not do this by yourself, but seek direction from your doctor or nurse.

14. Why every four hours? Wouldn't it make more sense if I just take the morphine when the pain begins to come back?

During recent days or weeks, your pain has proved to be persistent. It may be relieved completely by the recommended dose of morphine but, unfortunately, your pain is going to come back after several hours unless more medication is taken. Think of a similar situation: people with diabetes do not wait until they feel loaded with sugar and unwell before they take their next dose of insulin. With the help of a doctor or nurse they work out how much insulin they need in twenty-four hours to keep things balanced. This is what we aim to do when we treat your pain.

Starting Treatment With Morphine

With morphine in solution, experience has shown that 'every four hours' gives the best combination of good pain relief and least side effects in almost all patients. Very elderly patients (85+) and those with poor kidneys may well be able to take it less often.

If you take morphine just 'as needed', you are prescribing yourself alternating periods of comfort and pain – because the pain has to return before the next dose is taken. The next dose will take up to 30–40 minutes to ease the pain again. That could mean a total of, say, one hour of pain out of every four or five. As this is avoidable pain, it seems crazy to handle things that way. With morphine in solution, *regularly every four hours* is the recipe for good round-the-clock relief.

15. What should I do if I get behind with my medication?

In hospital, it should be possible to be fairly precise about 'every four hours' – 2 a.m., 6 a.m., 10 a.m., 2 p.m., 6 p.m., and 10 p.m. Though, sometimes, nursing restrictions can make the theoretical ideal more difficult to achieve than at home. In practice, most patients do not wake up on the dot of 6 a.m. In consequence, we recommend that 6 a.m. is interpreted as 'on waking', unless you happen to wake, say, after 8 a.m. This means that the 6 a.m. dose might not be taken until 6.30, 7 a.m., or even later. Even so, the next dose should be taken at 10 a.m., and then by the clock for the rest of the day. In short, *if you get behind, catch up at the next dose.* If you delay, you may find you have difficulty remembering a different time schedule every day. 'On waking, 10 a.m., 2 p.m., 6 p.m.' is easy to handle because it is easy to remember.

At 10 p.m. the same flexibility may be necessary as at 6 a.m. Some patients find that they need to go to bed at, say, 9 p.m. and they are fast asleep by 10 p.m. For this reason, it is best for most patients to regard 10 p.m. and 'at bedtime' as interchangeable. Obviously, if your day does not start till 9 a.m. and you never go to bed until midnight, a more individual timetable may be necessary – but the principle of every four hours by the clock remains the same.

Oral Morphine

16. How soon will I become pain-free?

If you have many pains, and if you are depressed or very anxious, it may take three to four weeks to achieve maximum relief.

Immediate total success is a bonus. The first goal will be to get you a good night's sleep and to make you more comfortable during the day. The second goal is complete relief at rest during the day. The final goal is freedom from pain when walking and moving around. This third level of pain control is not always possible with drugs alone, and some people may need to limit certain activities if they find that these continue to bring on pain.

17. What about the nights? Do I need to set my alarm clock for 2 a.m.?

In theory 'Yes', but in practice the answer is frequently 'No'. If you are elderly and are in the habit of waking in the middle of the night to empty your bladder, a 2 a.m. dose can easily be included. In this case, after you take your 10 p.m./bedtime dose, measure out the 2 a.m. dose into the medicine cup and leave it beside the bed for when you wake. If you are half-asleep when you respond to the call of nature, you won't have to fumble around trying to measure out the correct dose. This can be doubly difficult on a cold and dark winter's night. It also means you will be less likely to disturb your partner.

If you wake again later in the night, the empty medicine cup will tell you that you have already had your 2 a.m. dose, and that all will be well until the morning. There will be no need to rack your brain trying to remember whether or not you have had your middle-of-the-night dose. As with 6 a.m. and 10 p.m., you can be flexible. If you wake to empty your bladder at 1 a.m. – take the 2 a.m. medicine then. If you wake free of pain at 3 a.m. – take it then.

On the other hand, if you do not regularly wake to empty your bladder during the night, there is probably no need to take a 2 a.m. dose. The reason for this is explained in the next section.

18. A double dose at bedtime? Isn't that a bit dangerous?

Most patients get through the night without a 2 a.m. dose provided they take a double dose at bedtime. (Sometimes in the elderly, one

Starting Treatment With Morphine

and a half times the normal daytime dose is enough.) Unbroken nights, both for you and the family, are a bonus to good pain control.

By giving a double dose at bedtime, the amount of morphine in the blood will be much higher, and this will cause drowsiness. While this is a disadvantage during the day, it is an advantage at night. By the morning, the amount of morphine in the blood will be back to usual levels prior to the first daytime dose.

We have information on file to show that a double dose at bedtime is effective through the night and that it is no more risky or dangerous than a single dose at 10 p.m. and another at 2 a.m. For most patients, therefore, 'every four hours', means 'on waking, 10 a.m., 2 p.m., 6 p.m., and a double dose at bedtime.'

19. Why do I have to take it so often? Couldn't I have a stronger mixture and take it less often?

A larger dose would be effective for longer but there would be a greater chance of troublesome side effects. Every four hours gives the best combination of good pain relief and least side effects.

Long-acting tablets are available and are particularly suitable for patients on a steady dose. These usually need to be taken only every 12 hours. If the dose does not maintain a satisfactory level of comfort, the dose should be increased rather than taking the tablets more often. Occasionally it is necessary to take the tablets every 8 hours. To take a long-acting drug more frequently than this would, however, defeat the purpose of such a preparation.

20. Will I need to use other pain relief drugs with morphine?

Many patients do, though not all. You may need aspirin or a similar drug. Morphine and aspirin together are particularly effective in bone pain. Morphine acts on pain centres in the brain and spinal cord, while aspirin acts more locally where you are having the pain.

Cortisone and related drugs are of benefit for certain types of cancer pain, particularly neuralgia. A variety of other 'helper' drugs may be recommended by your doctor. For example, if your pain is partly caused by muscle spasm, it will be helped by a muscle relaxant.

Oral Morphine

21. What will happen to me if morphine does not relieve my pain?

Treatments for cancer pain can be grouped under two broad headings:
- Pain relief drugs.
- Non-drug treatments.

Morphine is one of a range of useful and important pain relief drugs. In practice (and quoting the World Health Organisation again), *drugs usually give good relief provided the right drug is taken in the right dose at the right time intervals.*

The more important non-drug treatments are:
- Psychological support for you and your family.
- Limiting certain activities (if pain is made worse by them).
- Radiation therapy (particularly for pain in bones).
- Injections to deaden nerves (useful in a small number of cases).

Psychological treatments such as relaxation therapy are helpful for many patients.

22. Does it matter when I take the morphine in relation to my meals?

No. The times that people eat vary. We have never had to take this into account in patients prescribed oral morphine.

23. Is there anything I can add to make the morphine solution taste better?

Unflavoured morphine sulphate solutions taste bitter. While some patients do not mind this (or may even like it), most people find the bitterness unpleasant. Pouring the required amount of morphine into a medicine cup and adding milk, orange or other juice is the solution favoured by many.

Many pharmacies have a flavoured base to which the morphine is added. In other words, the morphine is supplied with a flavour included, and is usually sweetened. Some patients, however, find the sweetness less acceptable than the original bitterness.

Starting Treatment With Morphine

24. Will I be able to drive the car if I am taking morphine?

Doctors have a legal responsibility to advise patients if a disability is likely to make them a danger when driving. There is an obligation on the driver to report any such disability to the licensing authority, unless relatively short-term (e.g. less than three months).

Taking morphine for medicinal reasons does *not* automatically disqualify you from driving. Your general alertness and reaction time may, however, be affected by your medication.

It is important that you take the following precautions, particularly if you have not driven for some weeks because of ill health:
- Do not drive in the dark or when conditions are bad.
- Do not drink alcohol, however little, during the day.
- Check your fitness to drive in the following way:
  – Choose a quiet time of the day when the light is good.
  – Choose an area where there are a number of quiet roads.
  – Take a companion (husband, wife, friend).
  – Drive for 10–15 minutes on quiet roads.
  – If both you and your companion are happy with your alertness, concentration, reactions and general ability, then it is all right to drive for short distances.
- Do not exhaust yourself by long journeys.

It is perhaps worth pointing out that many patients receiving morphine are not well enough to drive, and have no wish to do so. To drive or not to drive is perhaps an issue only for a minority.

WORKING THROUGH ANY UNWANTED SIDE EFFECTS

25. Doesn't morphine have a lot of side effects?

The common side effects seen with morphine therapy are:

At the beginning
- Vomiting.
- Drowsiness.
- Unsteadiness.
- Confusion.

Continuing
- Constipation.

Occasional
- Sweating.

Note: Respiratory depression and 'addiction' are *not* listed.

Although this may at first seem a disturbing list, it is important to emphasize that *it is rare* for treatment with oral morphine to be abandoned because of side effects. Usually, the early side effects ease with time or an antidote is available. These issues are discussed further in the following sections.

26. Will I need medication to counteract nausea and vomiting?

If you vomit after taking your medication, the morphine will not be absorbed from the gut, the pain will continue, and you will lose confidence in the new medicine. To avoid this, some doctors recommend the routine use of an anti-vomiting drug when morphine is prescribed. Others prescribe for selected patients only.

You will certainly need to take an anti-vomiting drug if:
- You are already troubled by nausea and vomiting.
- You are vomiting as a result of taking codeine or one of its alternatives.
- You have vomited with morphine and similar drugs in the past.

You probably will not need an antivomiting drug if:
- You have no nausea and vomiting at the moment.
- You have already taken codeine or another morphine-like drug regularly without nausea and vomiting.

One-third of all patients prescribed morphine never need an anti-vomiting drug.

Working Through Any Unwanted Effects

27. Will I have to go on taking the anti-vomiting drugs?

Vomiting with morphine is sometimes just an early side effect. Your doctor may, therefore, reduce the dose of the anti-vomiting drug or phase it out altogether. This may be done after you have been on a steady dose of morphine for one to two weeks. If the nausea returns, this is likely to be a sign that you need to stay on an anti-vomiting drug.

28. Will I get drowsy on morphine?

Like vomiting, drowsiness tends to be troublesome particularly during the first few days, possibly up to a week. It might come back again if the dose of morphine is increased. You should persevere in the knowledge that the drowsiness will lessen after a few days.

Occasionally, in the very old and frail, it is necessary to reduce the dose of morphine and then increase it again more slowly, every 2–3 days, until adequate pain relief is obtained.

29. Will I go on feeling drowsy or drugged?

Occasionally, yes. It is important to distinguish between persistent drowsiness and inactivity drowsiness. Most patients receiving morphine 'catnap' with ease. This means that you may drop off to sleep if sitting quietly and alone. This can be an advantage if you have limited stamina and require more rest and sleep than you did before you developed cancer. On the other hand, if your stamina is not greatly limited, you will find that you can live a relatively normal life.

If your work demands long hours at a desk, you may find you cannot concentrate for long and tend to sleep. If this happens, a trial of a brain stimulant may be indicated. Other causes of drowsiness should, however, first be excluded by your doctor – particularly sedative drugs or certain sleeping tablets which take a long time to be cleared out of the body.

Oral Morphine

30. Will I get confused?

If you are over 70, you may become muddled at times during the first few days of treatment with morphine, but persevere – your mind will clear.

31. Will I get dizzy?

Again, those over 70 may experience dizziness or feel unsteady for a few days. You should continue with the morphine knowing that this unpleasant sensation will subside as your body adjusts to the morphine.

32. What about constipation?

This is the most troublesome side effect of treatment with morphine, and other strong pain-killers. It is important that you seek suitable advice from your doctor about laxatives and learn to manage your bowels effectively.

Do not stop taking the morphine even if controlling the constipation proves more difficult than controlling the pain.

Ask your doctor to prescribe an appropriate laxative when the morphine is started. Your doctor may prescribe both a softener and a stimulant laxative. These are available in combined as well as in separate preparations. The following should be noted:
- You do not need a bowel movement every day.
- Aim for a bowel movement every second or third day; more is a bonus.
- If you have no bowel movement for three days, use a suppository or arrange for an enema to be given by a nurse.
- Drink plenty of fluids.
- Prune juice can help in the mornings.
- If you are eating well and have a good appetite, increase dietary fibre by adding bran to your breakfast cereal, or use a bulk laxative regularly every day.
- If your appetite is poor, do not force yourself to eat fibre.

Working Through Any Unwanted Effects

33. I find I've been sweating a lot since I started the morphine. Is this connected?

Some patients complain of sweating. This can be heavy, and tends to be more marked at night. Sweating may also be troublesome if you have a fever. Sleep in thin nightclothes and in a cool room with a change of clothes near at hand.

Sometimes cortisone is of benefit. You might like to discuss this with your doctor.

34. What happens if I am allergic to morphine?

Don't worry, you won't be! Perhaps one person in a thousand complains of itching with oral morphine therapy. A change may be needed to one of the alternatives to morphine (e.g. phenazocine, levorphanol, methadone).

In some patients, morphine slows down stomach emptying to such an extent that they feel nauseated, and may vomit, despite the use of one of the commonly prescribed anti-vomiting drugs. In this case, a change to an anti-vomiting drug that also hastens stomach emptying is indicated. This usually sorts the problem out. If not, it will be necessary to change from morphine to one of its alternatives.

On rare occasions only, patients taking morphine experience hallucinations, or have other disturbing psychological side effects. Such feelings may pass off spontaneously, or settle with a suitable antidote.

It is important to emphasize that a change from morphine to one of its alternatives is rarely necessary. Used carefully and under supervision, oral morphine has an excellent track record.

STILL MORE QUESTIONS ABOUT MORPHINE

35. Why morphine? I thought that was for pain, but my problem is shortness of breath.

If your breathing has become very rapid because of cancer affecting the lungs, morphine often helps by slowing the rate of breathing down. This makes you feel more comfortable. You are also less likely to end up gasping for breath when you get up and do things.

The reason morphine is often of benefit in this situation is that many of the extra breaths you are taking are not necessary for your system. An over-rapid rate of breathing tends to become inefficient. Slower and deeper breaths are of greater benefit.

The dose of morphine to reduce shortness of breath is usually smaller than those used to relieve pain. As always, the benefits must be weighed against the side effects. The aim of the morphine is to make you less short of breath and more relaxed. But, as with pain, morphine is not the cure-all for shortness of breath. If the shortness of breath relates to a second disorder such as asthma, bronchitis or heart failure, treatments other than morphine are more appropriate.

36. Is oral morphine really effective?

Yes. It is only rarely necessary to prescribe morphine by injection because oral morphine is not working.

37. Is it necessary to give more morphine by mouth than by injection?

Yes. As a general rule, the dose of morphine should be doubled when changing to the oral route. Occasionally it is necessary to increase this to three times the previously injected dose.

38. Wouldn't injections be better?

No. Oral medication results in a more constant drug level in the body. This leads to better pain relief and fewer side effects. Injections also tend to tie you to a second person unless you give your own.

Still More Questions About Morphine

39. Are injections ever needed?

Yes. Injections are necessary if you are:
- Vomiting a lot.
- Unable to swallow.

Once the vomiting has been controlled using an anti-vomiting drug (also by injection), it is often possible to go back to giving the medicines by mouth.

40. Once on injections, is it possible to change successfully to the oral route?

Yes, though it is often wise to convert to the oral route in stages. For example, the anti-vomiting drug can be changed first, followed the next day by the 10 a.m. and 6 p.m. dose of morphine. Finally, the other doses can be changed. The 'run-in' period with the other medication gives guidance as to whether oral administration is going to be successful.

A progressive conversion may also be necessary if you find it difficult to believe that oral medication will be as effective.

41. Can morphine be given by suppository?

Yes. Suppositories of morphine sulphate are available in a number of strengths. They can also be made by a helpful pharmacist. The same amount is needed in suppositories as by mouth to control pain. Suppositories are a useful alternative to injections, particularly at home.

42. Why do some people need more morphine than others?

There are many reasons why this is so. These include:
- The cause of your pain.
- Differences in the severity of pain.
- Differences in sensitivity to pain.
- Differences in how the body uses morphine.
- Whether other pain relief drugs and/or non-drug measures are also being used.
- The presence or absence of other symptoms.

Oral Morphine

43. What about the Brompton cocktail?

This is a traditional mixture of morphine and cocaine in a base of syrup, alcohol and chloroform water. It offers no advantages over a simple solution of morphine sulphate in water. In addition, it causes more side effects. It is more nauseating (due to the syrup content) and may cause a burning sensation in the throat (due to the alcohol).

44. Is diamorphine (heroin) better than morphine?

By mouth, morphine and diamorphine have similar actions and unwanted effects. By the time diamorphine reaches the brain it has been converted by the body to morphine. Thus, when given by mouth, diamorphine should be considered as just an alternative way of getting morphine to the pain centres of the brain and spinal cord.

45. Why do they create such a fuss about giving morphine in hospital? If there is only one registered nurse on duty, I often have to wait ages until one comes from the next ward.

The apparent fuss relates to legal requirements. Certain drugs, morphine included, are 'scheduled' or 'controlled'. This means double-checking and more careful book-keeping – hence the second nurse. The idea behind the regulations is to prevent drugs which are attractive to addicts from getting into the wrong hands. The regulations are *not* intended to prevent cancer patients from receiving an adequate quantity of morphine. It is obviously upsetting if a shortage of nurses has this effect.

QUESTIONS FROM A RELATIVE OR CLOSE FRIEND

46. Will it say on the bottle that it's morphine?

The bottle may be clearly labelled 'morphine', or it may simply be called by a brand name. We, however, see no reason for secrecy. In fact, we would discourage it. The reason for secrecy is fear. This false fear is based on false ideas of what morphine is and does.

It often gives people a mental jolt when they learn that morphine is being prescribed. A few days later, though, most patients are very pleased to be taking it – because of greatly improved comfort. As they are more comfortable and sleeping better, they have a renewed interest in life. These and other positives soon outweigh any possible negatives.

Some patients need morphine, either continuously or periodically, for several months or years. To commence morphine does not necessarily mean someone is close to death. Rather, it means that the patient has a severe pain that requires something stronger than codeine.

47. Is it necessary to keep the morphine locked up?

It is almost unheard of for patients to have an oral solution of morphine stolen by family, friends or intruders. However, as with all medicines, it is advisable to keep morphine out of sight and in a cupboard where young children cannot reach it.

48. Is it all right to keep the bottle of morphine with the other medicines?

Yes. Morphine solutions almost always have a preservative in them to prevent fungi and yeasts from growing in them. Though, in very hot weather, it may be best to keep the morphine in a refrigerator.

Oral Morphine

49. Will the morphine mix all right with his other medicines?

It is usually best to link all the patient's medicines to the times that the morphine is taken. Thus a heart tablet taken once a day can be linked with either 6 a.m. or 10 a.m. Laxatives, too, can often be linked with the bedtime morphine. Other tablets may be linked with 10 a.m. and bedtime, or 10 a.m., 2 p.m., and 6 p.m. This will depend on how many times a day the tablets have to be taken, and whether they have to be spaced out around the clock, or whatever.

Occasionally, because morphine delays stomach emptying in some patients, the combination of morphine and, for example, cortisone may result in acid indigestion, whereas either alone would not. Similarly, the combined use of morphine and certain tranquilizers may together cause troublesome drowsiness, whereas either alone does not. Provided the doctor is alert to such possibilities, the necessary corrective action can be taken. We nevertheless emphasize that, generally speaking, morphine can be given (and taken) in combination with virtually all types of other medication.

50. Since he has had the pain his appetite has gone completely. Will the morphine help him to eat better?

Many people lose interest in eating and in life generally if their whole horizon becomes one of severe never-ending pain. This is particularly so if sleep has been disturbed and the patient is exhausted both physically and mentally. In these circumstances, better pain control and adequate sleep is likely to result in a renewed interest in eating.

On the other hand, there are many reasons for loss of appetite in cancer. This means that, if he continues to be disinterested in food despite good pain control, the doctor will have to look at the problem as a separate issue. Nausea and severe constipation are two relatively common causes of loss of appetite.

51. Will she be safe looking after the baby if she is taking morphine?

Breast-feeding is not possible if the mother is taking morphine, because some of the morphine will be transferred to the child in the mother's milk. This question usually refers to a toddler rather than a

Questions From a Relative or Close Friend

baby-in-arms. Here, the answer depends on the mother's general stamina more than anything else. Most mothers in this position find the incessant demands of a pre-school child very difficult to cope with, and some kind of child-minding has to be arranged.

In short, within the limits of her stamina, there is no reason why a mother taking morphine should be discouraged from caring for her child. Indeed, as she will be more comfortable and sleeping well, someone on morphine is likely to cope better than would otherwise be the case.

52. What about signing legal documents while taking morphine?

It all depends on the patient's general circumstances. For many patients, the use of morphine brings about a welcome improvement in their general condition. There will also be some who are too ill to sign such documents whether or not they are taking morphine. For those who become very drowsy or muddled when starting morphine, it makes good sense to delay signing important documents for a few days. By doing this, it will be difficult for someone at a later date to cast doubt on the patient's ability to think clearly at the time of signing.

53. What should I do if he insists on having more than he has been prescribed? Could it kill him?

If left to their own devices, patients are more likely to take too little rather than too much. Assuming that the reason for more morphine is to relieve distressing pain, there are no grounds for refusing the request. Obviously, if more than a double or treble dose is insisted on, there may have to be a certain resistance:

'I'll give you a double dose now, and then ring Dr X. to let him know the prescribed dose is not holding the pain. If he says to give more, or repeat a double dose after an hour or so, that's fine. I just think we need more guidance.'

Should the patient receive too much, it will most probably act like the bedtime double dose (see Section 18). The patient will sleep for several hours and, with luck, will wake refreshed and free of pain.

Oral Morphine

54. Is there a danger that she will use the morphine to commit suicide?

The incidence of suicide in cancer patients is no greater than in the general population. Some cancer patients, if caught up in a living hell of unrelieved pain, think of killing themselves. Surprisingly few do. In our experience, when the pain is relieved – often with morphine – the patient no longer thinks of suicide. Moreover, out of several thousand cancer patients, we know of no one who has used a solution of morphine to attempt suicide.

55. If he has no pain and refuses to take the next dose, do I insist on him taking it?

It depends on the circumstances. If the patient is totally confused, the refusal may be unreasonable. In this case, continued pressure to accept the morphine may be necessary. On the other hand, if the confusion is associated with paranoia (feelings of being threatened or persecuted), even gentle persuasion might make matters worse. If in doubt, don't – and seek help from your doctor or visiting nurse, possibly by phone in the first instance.

If misunderstanding due to confusion is not the cause, he will presumably have a reason for declining the medication. He may be right: it does cause unacceptable drowsiness or nausea in his case. Or perhaps the untreated constipation is merely exchanging one hell for another. There is obviously room for exploring the reason or reasons behind the refusal. Here too, professional advice should be sought.

56. If she becomes unconscious, should the morphine be discontinued?

No. Mainly for two reasons:
- Unconscious patients in pain tend to become restless.
- Physical dependence usually develops after several weeks of oral morphine therapy. If this is the case, and the morphine is stopped abruptly, the patient is even more likely to become restless.

If the degree of physical dependence is considerable, she might also start to sweat a lot and might possibly develop uncontrolled diarrhoea.

A BROADER VIEW

Pain is not a simple sensation like seeing or hearing: it is far more complex. Several thousand years ago, Aristotle described it as 'a passion of the soul'. It certainly reflects a major area of body-mind interaction. Intensity of pain is modified not only by medication but also by mood, morale and the meaning of the pain to us as individuals. Living with cancer is hard work and there are often plenty of negative factors to contend with – loss of energy, loss of job and financial independence, and so on. All these factors, and more, influence how sensitive we are to any underlying physical pain sensations. We have tried to put these ideas together in the following diagram:

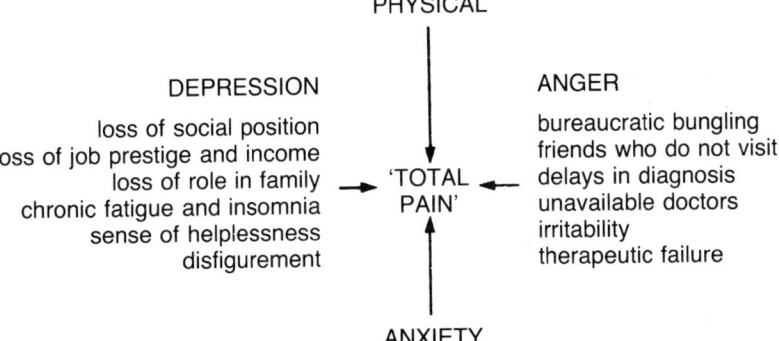

Oral Morphine

When pain is seen in this way it explains why the companionship and support of your family and friends are so important to you at this time. Equally important is the ongoing support of an attentive doctor and of the hospital or visiting nurses. They are just as necessary as the right pain relief medication. The two work together; either alone is not enough.

USEFUL ADDRESSES

If you feel you need more help than you are currently getting, you might like to telephone or write to one of the following addresses.

BACUP
121–123 Charterhouse Street
London EC1M 6AA
Tel: 01-608 1661

Cancer Relief Macmillan Fund
Anchor House
15–19 Britten Street
London SW3 3TZ
Tel: 01-351 7811

CancerLink
46a Pentonville Road
London N1 9HF
Tel: 01-833 2451

Help The Hospices
BMA House
Tavistock Square
London WC1H 9JP
Tel: 01-388 7807

Marie Curie Memorial Foundation
28 Belgrave Square
London SW1X 8QG
Tel: 01-235 3325